HOW TO RECOGNIZE MENTAL ILLNESS IN YOUTH

and When to Start Intervention

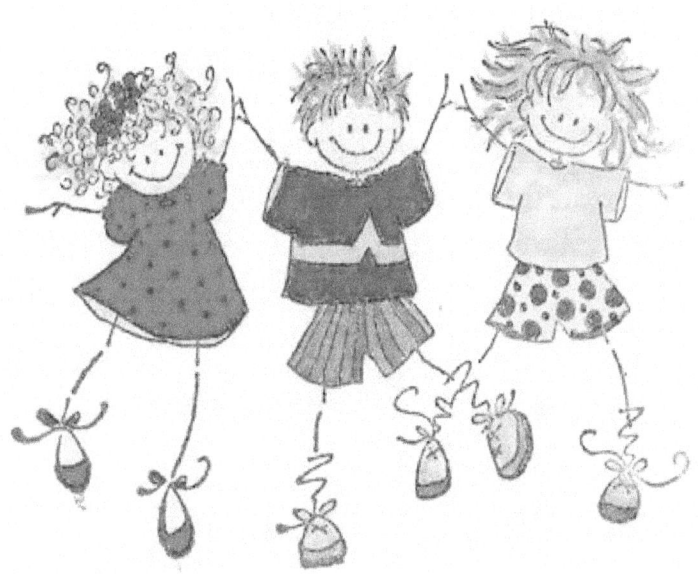

By Patricia A. Carlisle

Introduction

I want to thank you and congratulate you for choosing the book, *"HOW TO RECOGNIZE MENTAL ILLNESS IN YOUTH AND WHEN TO START INTERVENTION"*.

This book contains proven steps and strategies on how to recognize the symptoms in youth and understand when to seek treatment.

Mental illness can only be diagnosed by a professional. However, this does not mean you cannot take notice of some warning signs. If the problem is discovered in time, you can treat and keep it under control with the right treatment. This is especially true for mental illness in youth. The sooner a doctor diagnoses the problem, the more chances there are for treating it. Some of these signs can seem normal at first glance. All teenagers present these symptoms sometimes.

However, it is important to reach deeper into the issue.

Thanks again for choosing this book, I hope you enjoy it!

Patricia A. Carlisle, MSW, CBT

Patricia Carlisle- A Master Social Worker and a Cognitive Behavioral Therapist (CBT) gives out an expression of how important it is for an individual to take into consideration the concept of self-assessment to know what human, technical and conceptual skills they posses to perform or to achieve what they desire, or to deal with everyday life. However, every particular group of people has their own unique set of ideas, traditions and events including the frame of mind according to which people perform but there are many who faces problems and fail to maintain a healthy mind set affecting their behaviors and performance to those around them.

> People like Patricia Carlisle are among those who have felt this urge of serving people and helping them out of their mental crisis towards a healthy life. She has experienced some close encounters in her personal life regarding mental health issues in her family and friends that has encouraged her to pursue this as her career.

Currently Patricia Carlisle is serving as a Certified On-Line Cognitive Behavioral Therapist with an extensive 15years of experience using Cognitive-Behavior Therapy Techniques. She envisions a world where everyone gets mental health treatment with no mental health stigma and to make it real she has already set up her own Holistic Measure Online Comprehensive Behavioral Healthcare Company after retiring from The Nord Center in The Partial Hospitalization Program (PHP) Dept for 5 years and Murtis H. Taylor Mental Health Center as a mental health counselor, psychological support technician and case manager for 10 years to emulsify her skills more professionally. Along with this, she has wrote down her passion as a clinician in 25 or more short books to help individuals and families get their life back, freeing them of the restraints of negative thinking, anxiety and depression by using different approaches. She is highly appreciated among her clients for her flexibility and professionalism of dealing with them graciously.

To reach her, make use of her direct website address: http://therapist2013.wix.com/e-therapy . As she is ready to inspire hope and contribute to health and well-being by providing the best online health care through comprehensive practice, education and research.

TABLE OF CONTENT

Chapter 1

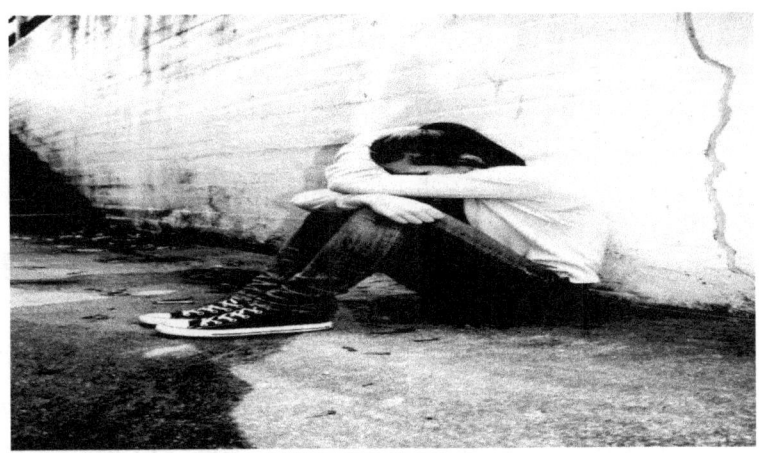

DEPRESSION

One of the most common signs of mental illness in young people is prolonged depression. Is your teenager locked up in his or her room for hours and always seems sad? He or she might also refuse to talk to you or anyone else. There might be a good reason for this. Try to talk to him and find out if something happened at school or with his friends. If he has no real reason for his depression, you might consider this as a warning sign.

Some teenagers just want to be alone to chat online with their friends or talk on the phone. They might also be going through a bad breakup. Remember that first love in youth is very intense. They can also see everything as a drama. If that is the case, you have no reason to worry. This is absolutely normal, however, if your teenager just wants to be alone and has no contact with his or her friends, you need to take this seriously.

Depression can be in the form of deep sadness and isolation, or it can manifest with strong feelings of anger. If you cannot make him or her open up to you, it's time to ask for help from a doctor. Even if you are wrong about it, it is always better to be safe than sorry. Until you can get help, try to distract him or her with things you know they love.

For example, you can find that new video game he or she was asking for or you can go watch a funny movie together. Another good idea is to organize a party. This is a good method to help your teenager make some friends. If all these things don't work, you should make an appointment with a professional right away.

Depression is a condition that needs urgent care. It is important to know that a person suffering with this doesn't necessarily have a reason for it. If it's real depression you cannot fix it yourself with a night out or a good movie. In rare cases it can lead to suicide. This is why you should not wait for the person to recover by himself. He needs special medicines and therapy to successfully fight depression and win. The doctor's diagnosis might be that depression is connected to another mental illness.

Chapter 2

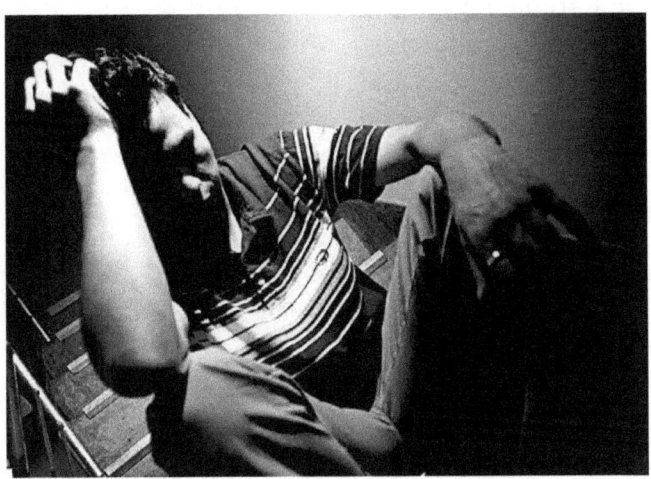

CONFUSED THINKING

Another big sign of mental illness in youth is confusion. Pay attention to see if you notice your teenager is often confused. For example he or she can forget what month it is or they may get lost on their way back home from school. If this happens only once or twice it does not mean anything. However, when this confusion is not just an isolated event, it's time to take action and start intervention. In some cases, the youth can end up not remembering who you are.

However, do not wait for this to happen in order to ask for help. Even little signs of continuous confusion can mean there is an underlining cause. If the youth shows confusion signs, pay attention to see if this becomes a pattern of behavior. It doesn't mean anything if it's just an isolated event. If you don't have the time to watch him yourself, ask the teacher to let you know if there are any signs of confusion during class.

Friends and other family members can also help. Be careful not to embarrass your teenager. You need to be discreet when you ask people to pay attention to this behavior. It is all for their own good but you should not make them feel self-conscious. In order to find the problem you need to allow the teenager to behave as he normally would.

Chapter 3

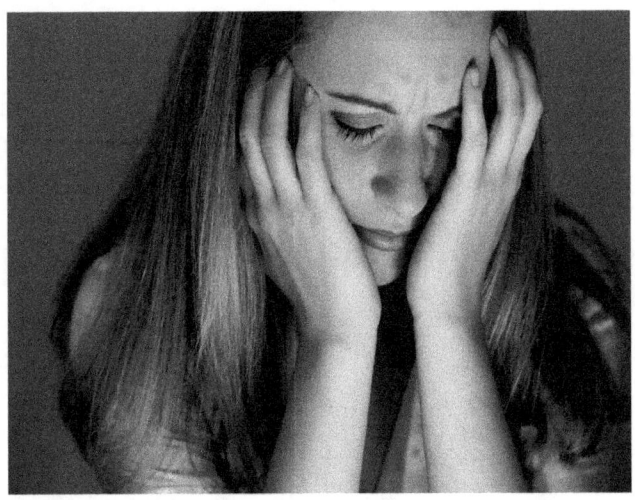

EXTREME HIGH AND LOWS

Extreme high and lows, also known as mood swings, are some other things you should look out for when trying to find warning signs of mental illness. This is when a teenager is acting very happy without a specific reason, only to change to the other extreme soon after. Teenagers are well known for temper tantrums. It is important not to confuse this with illness. You should start worrying when these high and lows are a common occurrence. Anybody can have a bad day but if it becomes a usual thing you need to wonder if this is a sign of something else. When in doubt, do not hesitate to call a professional. They are there to help you even if it is to answer your questions and put your mind at ease.

You might think that seeing a teenager happy can't be a negative thing. But imagine if he or she gets extremely happy out of the blue only to fall in deep sadness or anger minutes or hours later. This is when you need to ask yourself some questions. Hormonal changes in teenagers can also cause mood swings and this does not mean your child has a mental illness. This is only in the case when these mood swings are too extreme or they happen too often.

A common mental illness with these high and lows is called bipolar disorder. This is a very common illness and can be kept under control with treatment. It can be very difficult to deal with people suffering with this disorder. They can get really angry out of the blue and you need to learn how to handle it. Getting mad yourself as a response will not help. Try to keep your calm and understand that it is not their fault.

Chapter 4

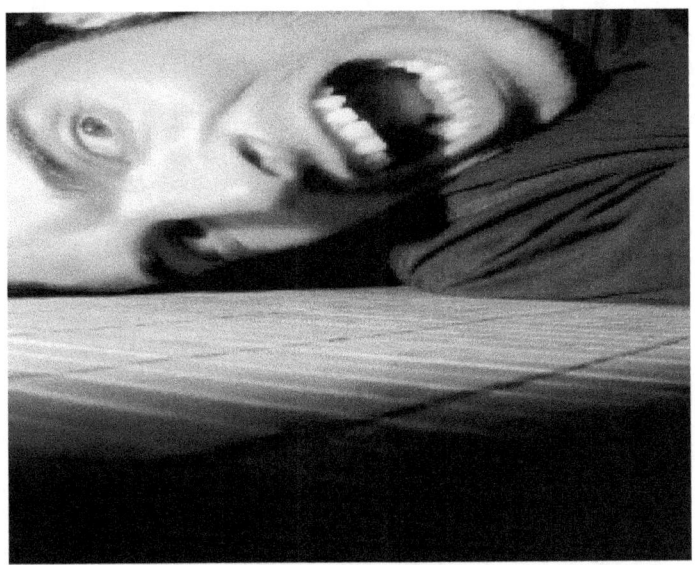

FEARS AND ANXIETIES

When young people have irrational fears and anxieties, you need to pay attention. Everybody is scared of one thing or another. However, if those fears take over one's life, this can mean a mental illness. In some rare cases, a person can refuse to leave the house because they are scared of something. Do not let it get to that. You can take charge of the situation and fix the problem in time.

As an example, most people are scared of spiders. They can scream, try to avoid them or even hide. This can be normal behavior. A warning sign is when a person is letting this fear affect his daily life. He can refuse to go to school or even outdoors because of this fear. The anxiety can be so powerful that it overpowers and stops them from having a normal life. It takes a lot of work and therapy to learn to control this fear. There are also a lot of anxiety medicines one can take to keep things under control and have a normal life.

The first step is to recognize there is a problem and talk to a doctor. A young person going through this might find it impossible to realize he or she has a real health problem. This is where family and friends come in play. It is usually easier to see the problem from the outside. The next step is to share your worries with the youth going through this.

Chapter 5

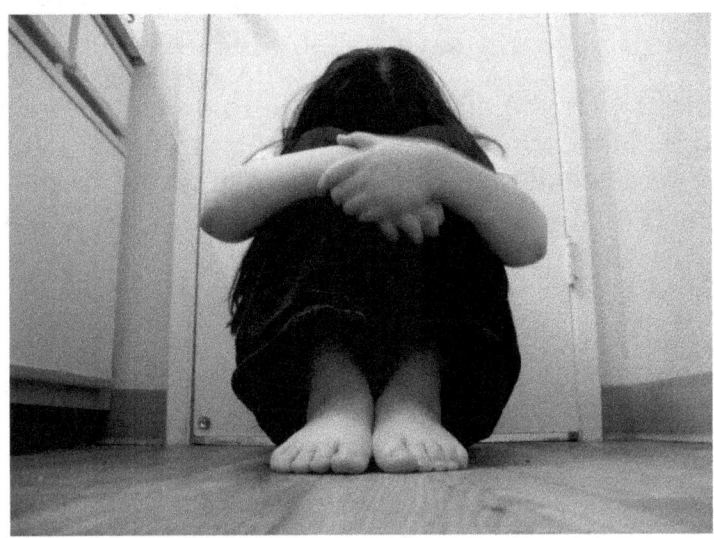

SOCIAL WITHDRAWAL

In the case of mental illness, young people have trouble coping with the outside world. They tend to want to be left alone and big crowds of people scare them. You will also notice that they have no friends at all. They prefer to spend their weekends inside the house, preferably in their bedroom. Whenever they are in public, they shut down and do not want to communicate. They are scared of big crowds and they can look like extremely shy people. In situations like this you need to look into it a little better. It might be something worse than just shyness.

Human beings are social by nature. It is healthy for us to be surrounded by other people, to have friends and communicate our feelings. This is why social isolation is not something to be taken lightly.

They also feel anxiety whenever they have to deal with other people. Speaking in public is out of question. However, many people are scared to speak in public. This can be normal. The social withdrawal has to be a lot more obvious than that. You will notice that they avoid parties and when they happen to go to one, they make absolutely no conversation with people. This can make it impossible for them to cope with the normal life. Going to school or having a job will be out of the question.

As a parent, you should not give into this. Do not allow your child to be homeschooled, have no friends and no job. Try to find the root problem for this social anxiety and fix it. Certain medicines and also talk therapy can make a real difference.

Chapter 6

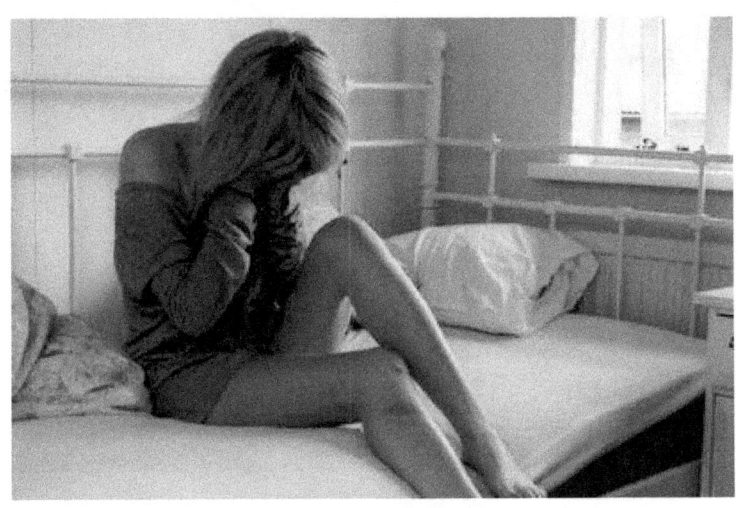

BIG CHANGES IN EATING AND SLEEPING BEHAVIOR

Any big change in a youth's life should be something to consider and looked into. This includes big changes in his eating or sleeping behavior. A young person suffering from a mental illness might suddenly lose their appetite and start suffering from sleep apnea. This can also be because of stress. This is why you need to communicate with him or her. Ask if there are any problems causing a lot of stress lately.

Maybe there are issues at school, with friends or maybe girlfriend/boyfriends problems. Whatever it is, if you find a good reason for these sudden changes, you can be relieved. Stress related problems are temporary. This means that as soon as what cause the problem disappears, everything will get back to normal. There is a real problem when you cannot find any apparent reason for the lack of appetite and sleep problems.

Chapter 7

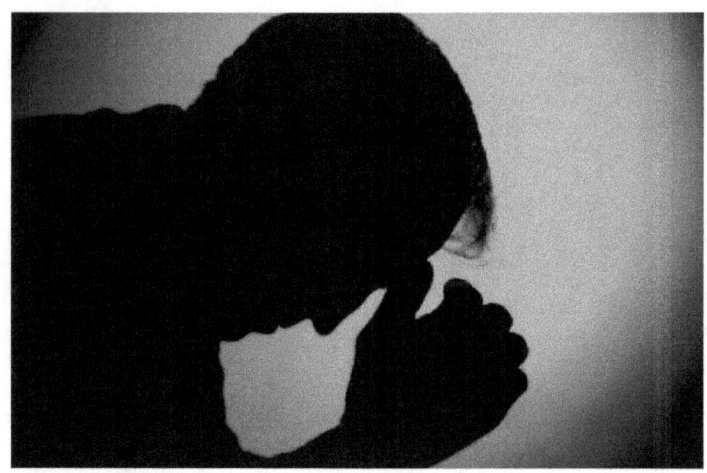

DELUSIONS OR HALLUCINATIONS

Delusions or hallucinations are clear signs of a mental illness. This is when someone starts believing things that makes no sense or starts seeing thing that aren't there. In this case there is absolutely no doubt that you need to ask for help from a doctor. These are warning signs of a more sever condition. You should not waste any time trying to guess what kind of illness this is. There are many types of mental illnesses and only a doctor can point you in the right direction for treatment. Hallucinations can lead to dangerous situations. If a teenager is showing these symptoms, he can harm himself or others. This is why, as parents you need to take action as soon as possible. Try not to let the situation get out of you control.

In some severe cases, parents aren't able to take care of the children suffering of delusions of hallucinations. This is very sad but sometimes it's better to allow people who know how to handle these illnesses take control.   This does not mean you are giving up on your child. It is quite the contrary. It takes a lot of courage to make a decision like this.

Chapter 8

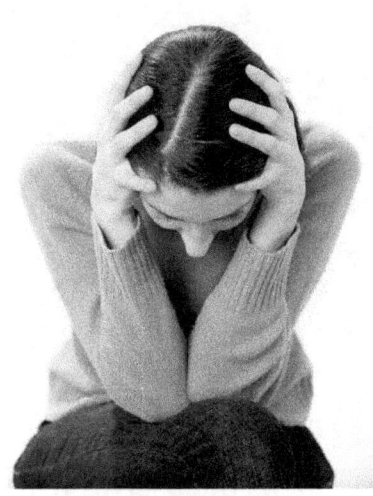

INABILITY TO COPE WITH DAILY ROUTINE

Simple tasks like doing homework, waking up early for classes, become impossible to do for young people suffering from a mental illness. They always seem like they are lost and it is almost impossible to focus. This alone however, is not a clear sign of mental illness. You need to check if there are other things that attract your attention such as confusion, delusions, hallucinations, or severe mood swings.

Do not take the inability to cope with daily tasks as the only sign of a mental illness. Sometimes it can be just a matter of laziness. Observe the youth for a few weeks and try to see if he or she is really trying. If they do all they can to cope with the routine and is unsuccessful, it is time to take action and check if the cause for this is a mental illness.

Chapter 9

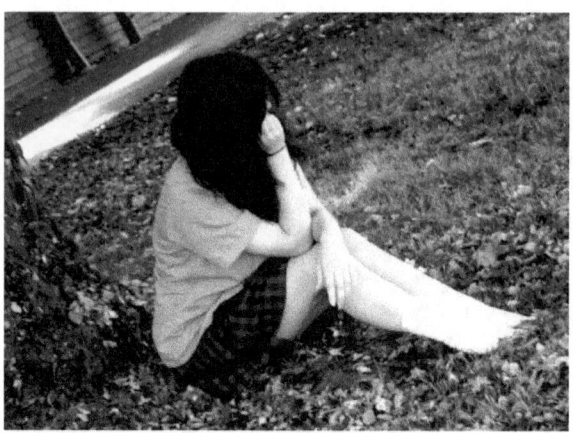

SUICIDAL THOUGHTS

If a young person threatens themselves with suicide, do not take it lightly. Even if it is just a way to attract attention, talking about death and suicide is never a good sign. This dark way of thinking might hide more than you can imagine. Suicidal thoughts can quickly become attempts to comment suicide.

There are things you can do to avoid this tragedy. Listen to him or her carefully. Sometimes he or she might not tell you exactly that they are thinking about committing suicide. They may only imply it or have a morbid fascination for death. It could be something like saying "I wish I was dead." People say things without meaning them all the time but it is better to take it seriously than regretting it later.

As you already know, teenagers are going through a lot of hormonal changes. They are also going through a transition period from childhood to adulthood. This can be very tough on some young people and can cause mental disturbances.

Chapter 10

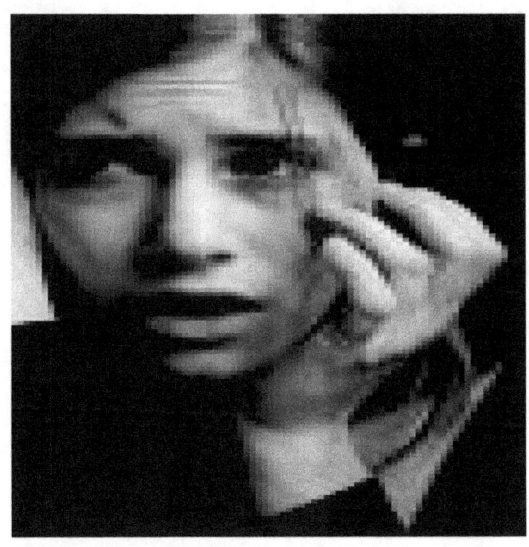

UNEXPLAINED PHYSICAL COMPLAINTS

If a young person is complaining all the time of physical illness and the doctor cannot really find the problem, this can be another sign of a mental illness. Before you reach this conclusion, make sure the physical complaints do not exist. Sometimes doctors can be wrong. This is why it is always good to ask for a second opinion.

The power of the mind is bigger than you think. If someone imagines a pain or illness, they will start to actually experience the symptoms even if they are physically healthy. They convince themselves they are ill. In reality the illness does exist but it is psychological.

Is your teenager feeling tired all the time even if he or she is getting enough sleep? This can be a sign of many illnesses but, one of them is mental illness. This is especially true when it comes to depression. One of the most common symptoms is the desire to sleep for a long time, even during the day. It is almost like they want to escape reality by sleeping and dreaming.

A mental illness puts a lot of stress on the body. This is why some unexplained physical symptoms may appear. For example, migraines are something a young person struggling with a mental illness might experience. Anxiety and fears can cause the body to react too. Some people will have stomach problems.

Chapter 11

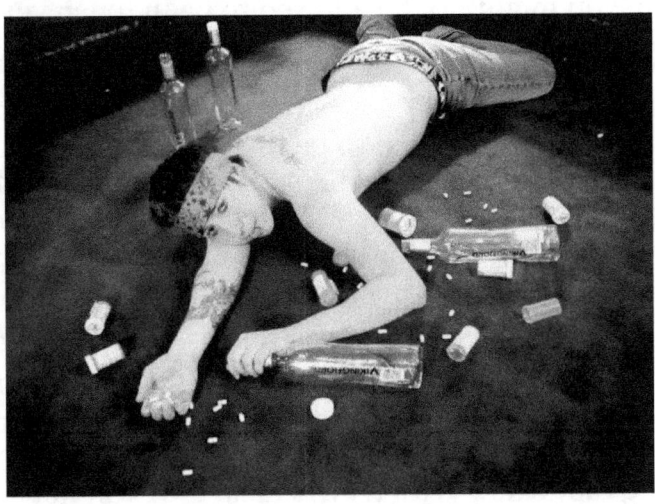

SUBSTANCE ABUSE

A teenager or a young person with a mental illness is more likely to start abusing drugs. This does not mean of course that every drug addict is also suffering from mental illness but it is very likely. The explanation for this is simple. Someone who is emotionally unstable can fall in the trap of addiction a lot easier than a healthy person. He or she might be looking for an escape. They find in drugs a way to get rid of their thoughts and feelings. Imagine being scared, stressed, or having delusions all the time. This can be very exhausting and this is why drugs seem like the best option.

If a young person started to abuse drugs, ask a doctor to make sure there is no psychological problem too. If he finds an illness, he or she will need double the help to treat the illness and the addiction. Each of these problems is a real challenge for any family.

However, do not lose hope. There is always a solution. Make sure you show him or her all your support. There are plenty of options. For example, you can ask your doctor for a referral. He can send you to a medical center where they specialize on drug addiction and mental illness. He or she might have to stay there for a couple of months. Depending on the condition, you might not be allowed to be in touch very much for the first month.

This can be very difficult on everyone involved. As a family member or friend, you need to be the strong one. Do not give up even if he or she accuses you of abandoning them there. When he or she is better they will realize that you did not just leave them there. It was for he or she own good and they will end up thanking you for this. Drug addicts will say things they don't really mean. Try not to let it affect you. That is not the real person talking. You need to understand and to forgive. When they recover from the addiction and taking the right treatment for the mental illness, he or she will regret everything they said. With a little luck, they will not even remember.

However, if he or she does, you need to make it clear that you forgave them. Guilt is another weight they do not need to carry around. This is how you can help. Make them understand it was not their fault at all. Show them how proud you are that he or she is on the right path. Having this kind of support from the people who love them are essential for recovery. It will give them the strength to keep on fighting.

Chapter 12

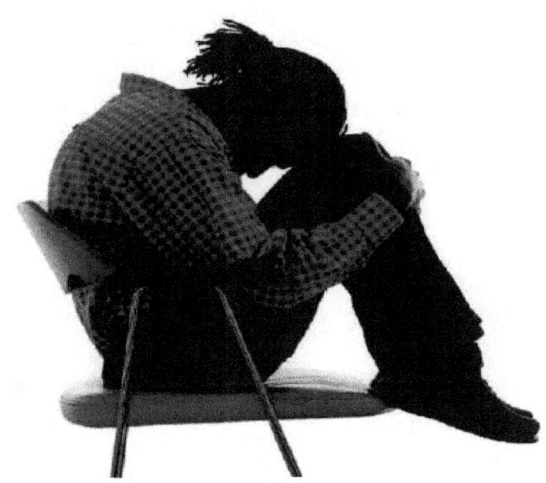

DEFIANCE OF AUTHORITY

Most young people will defy authority a few times. But when that defiance of authority becomes obvious, it is time to look into it. Does he or she have a reason for this? For example, if they really want to go to a party and as a parent you don't allow them, they might go anyway. This is okay. This is something we all did once or twice. Another reason they might be acting out is because of peer pressure. Check out their friends and see if they are a bad influence on them. You can also have the unpleasant surprise to find out that your child is the bad influence. As a parent, you tend to be on your child's side and think they are an angel being influenced by others. Try to keep a cool head and see things clearly.

However, if the defiance does not make any sense and they behave like this without an obvious reason, it can be a sign of a bigger mental health problem. He or she might be acting out at school and being rude to the teachers. If they are doing this with all the people that are supposed to be in charge, ask yourself why.

A reason more to worry is when there is a sudden change in the teenager's behavior. If before they use to be a child who was eager to please and never made any problems, you should find the reason why things are now different. The first step is to communicate with your youth. Find out if there are some things he or she didn't tell you about. There might be a logical explanation for their behavior towards authority lately. In situations like these, you need the professional opinion of a doctor.

Chapter 13

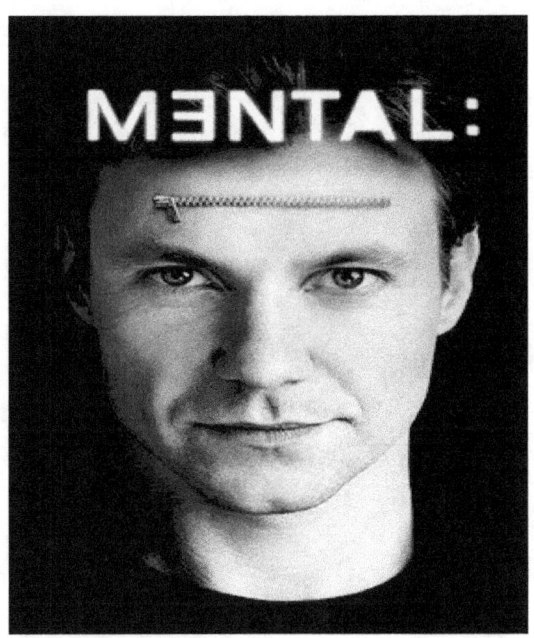

INABILITY TO MANAGE RESPONSIILITIES

Responsibilities and chores for the youth are not just a way to pass time. These tasks have an important role. A young person can learn how to manage responsibilities in life. This is what helps them grow up, learn work ethics, and form their personalities. When a teenager is unable to perform these simple daily chores, it can be a sign of a mental illness. If it is just about being lazy, it can be fixed with a good heart to heart talk.

However, you need to find out if there is something more there. Do you see him struggling to manage these responsibilities and fail? If he is trying his best and failing to perform, ask for the help of a professional.

Chapter 14

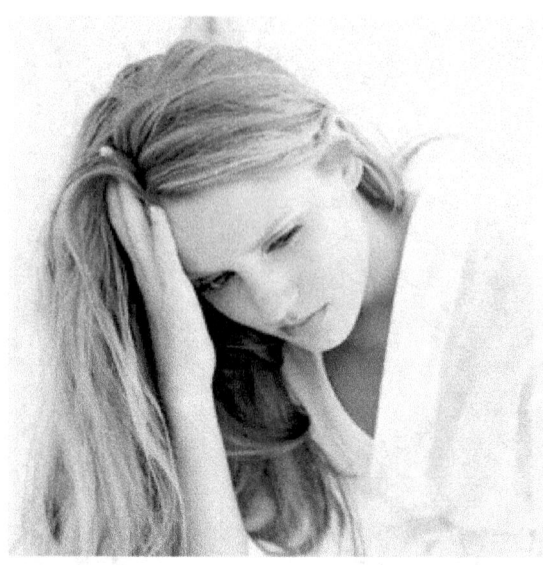

POOR GRADES

Poor grades happen because of two reasons. The young person is refusing to learn because he or she finds other fun things to do and they are simply lazy. Believe it or not, this is what you want. It is a lot easier to recover from laziness than from a mental illness.

One of the warning signs is when the teenager is easily distracted during class. He or she has difficulties focusing and paying attention to the teacher. Most of the time they are probably trying their best but it is impossible to keep up with their colleagues. This can be very frustrating and the child can end up feeling embarrassed. It is important to show your support and let them know that you know they are trying. Make a big deal whenever they are successful, no matter how small.

A specialist can find out if there is a mental problem and treat it. He or she might be offered private classes. In some cases, the best solution can be a special school. This will save them the frustration of always being behind their classmates. If he or she is staying in the same class and school, make sure you communicate to the teacher and diagnosis you get from the doctor. Try to always stay in touch so he can inform them about the progress they are making in class. Do not forget to praise them for every achievement. Every little success they have, takes a lot more effort than it would for a healthy teenager.

Chapter 15

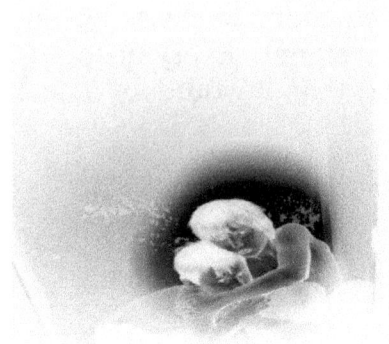

PERSISTENT NIGHTMARES

Is your child or youth always waking up in tears or screaming? Persistent nightmares can point to a possible mental illness.

If this situation continues, it is time to take action. A therapist can talk to him or her and find out the underlining cause. The nightmares can be only a symptom of the real issue. To make things easier for the child try to forbid them to watch violent horror movies or video games. This can be a trigger for bad dreams. A good night sleep is very important especially for young people who are still growing.

Chapter 16

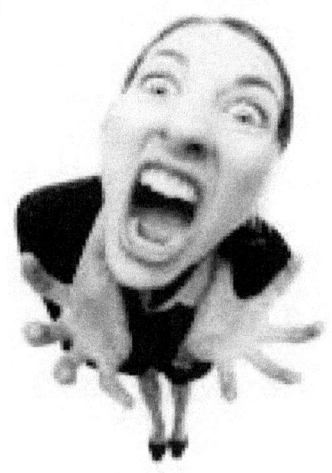

HYPERACTIVITY

Hyperactivity is something to worry about when it comes to a possible mental health problem. A young person might find it very difficult to sit in the same spot for more than a few minutes. He will also have difficulties paying attention or staying focused. A hyperactive person will talk very fast and change their idea in the middle of a sentence. Most of the times, they will make no sense at all. This is one case when it is recommended to start intervention.

Chapter 17

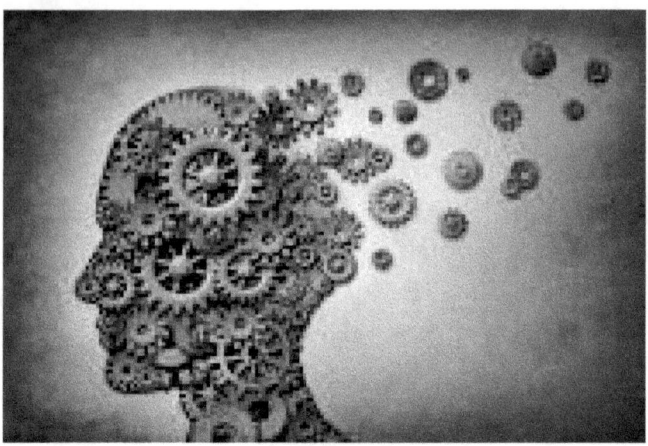

GETTING OVER A TRAUMA

If a young person went through something traumatic, he or she might be suffering from posttraumatic stress disorder. This is a normal reaction from a shock or trauma. It is treatable but is almost impossible to get over it without a doctor's help.

A trauma can cause other issues such as anxiety or depression. Even if a young person does not show any signs of posttraumatic stress disorder, it is recommendable to make sure by talking to a professional. Sometimes these signs show up much later when it might be too late or more difficult to treat.

These traumas can be very recent or can be from early childhood. Some people can keep things buried in their mind until they surface and cause problems. If this happens, talking to a therapist can be of great help. Adults find it difficult to get over traumas too but for the youth this can be even more difficult. They are already going through a lot of changes and their mind will not be able to cope with a trauma too. As an adult, if you know something happened, take action before there are any clear warnings.

__Conclusion__

Thank you again for choosing this book!

I hope this book was able to help you to become aware of the signs of mental illness in teens. Your job as the parent of a youth is to see the warning signs and alert a doctor. This is how you can help provide the right treatment in time and help your child get better. Mental illness in youth is more common than you think and you should not take it lightly.

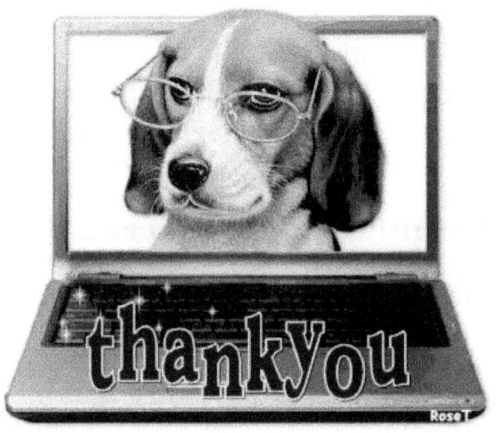

Finally, if you enjoyed this book, would you be kind enough to leave a review for this book on Amazon? It'd be greatly appreciated!

Thank you and good luck!

Preview Of 'MENTAL HEALTH STIGNMA: How to Overcome Mental health Stigma in America'

Chapter 1
DISCRIMINATION IMPACT OF STIGMAS

Stigma can prompt discrimination. Discrimination may be obvious and immediate, for example, someone making a negative comment about your mental illness or your treatment. On the other hand it might be unexpected or modest, for example, by keeping away from you because they expect you to be unsteady, savage or dangerous because of your mental health condition. You may start to judge yourself.

The destructive impact of stigma can include:

- Reluctance to look for help or treatment.

- Stop seeing family, friends, colleagues or others you know.

- Fewer doors open for employment, school, and social settings.

- Bullying, physical roughness or aggravation from others.

- Health insurance that doesn't cover your mental health treatment.

- The conviction that you'll never have the capacity to succeed at a specific tasks or that you can't improve your circumstances.

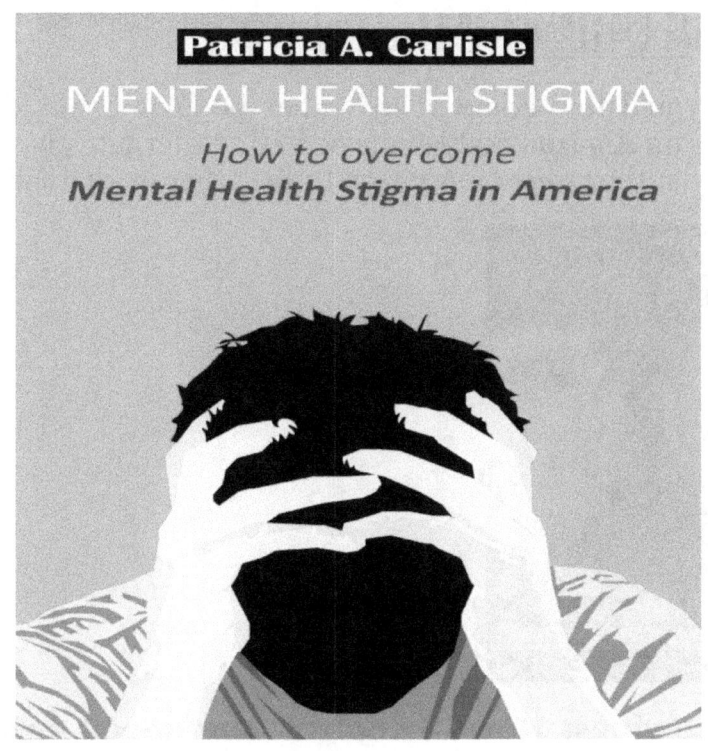

MENTAL HEALTH STIGMA: How to Overcome Mental Stigma in America.

Check Out My Other Books

Below you'll find some of my other popular books that are popular on Amazon and Kindle as well. Alternatively, you can visit my author page on Amazon to see other work done by me.

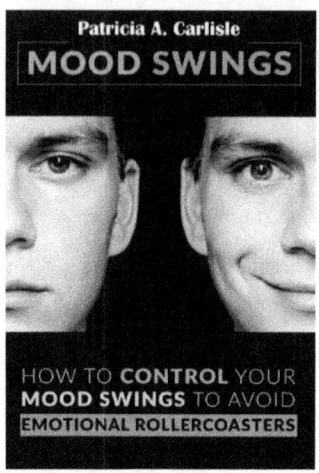

Mood Swings: How to control your mood swings to avoid emotional rollercoster's.

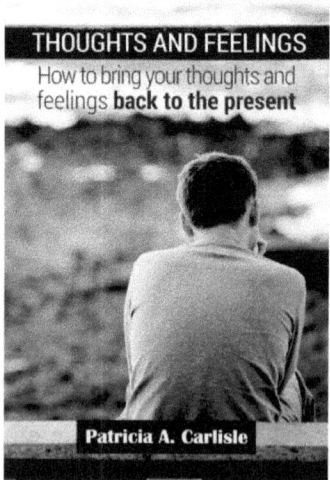

THOUGHTS AND FEELINGS: How to Bring Your thoughts and feelings back to the present.

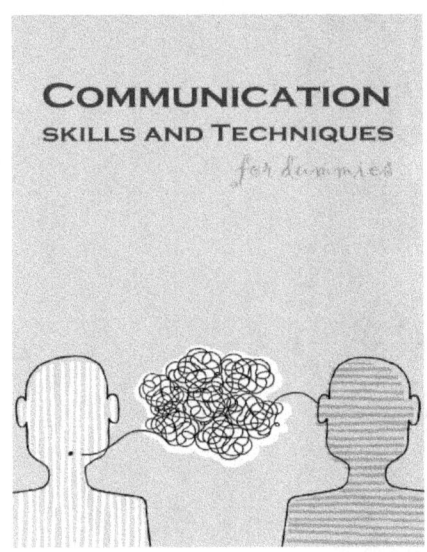

COMMUNICATION SKILLS AND TECHNIQUES FOR DUMMIES.

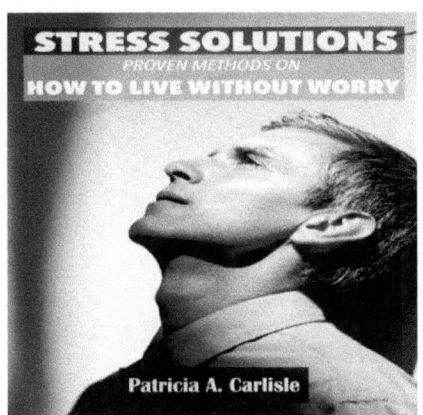

STRESS SOLUTIONS: Proven methods on how to live without worry.

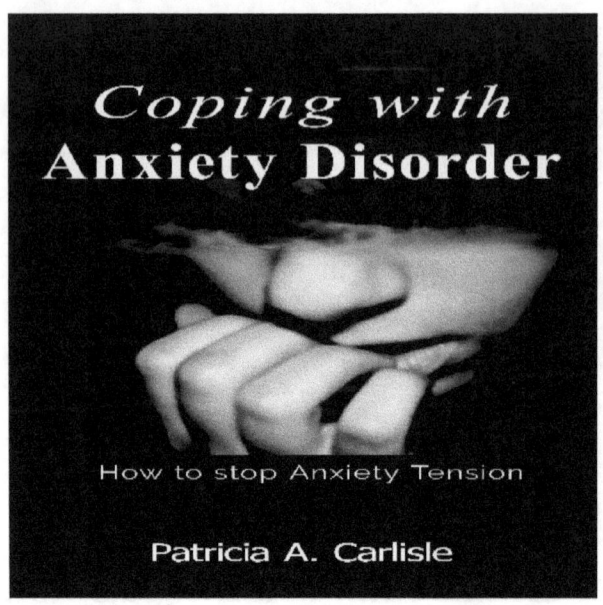

Coping with Anxiety Disorder: How to stop Anxiety Tension.

BONUS: SUBSCRIBE TO THE FREE BOOK

Beginners Guide to Yoga & Meditation

"Stressed out? Do You Feel Like The World Is Crashing Down Around You? Want To Take A Vacation That Will Relax Your Mind, Body And Spirit? Well this Easy To Read Step By Step

E-Book Makes It All Possible!"

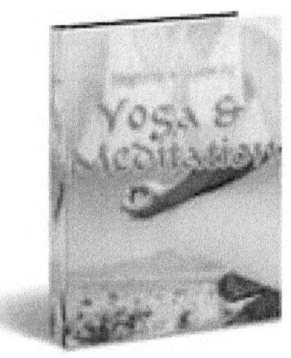

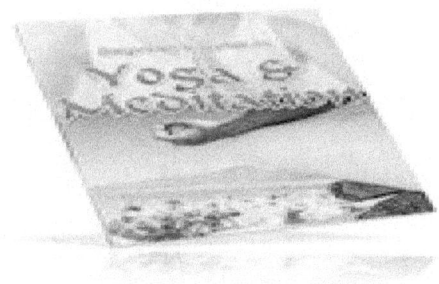

Instructions on how to join our mailing list, and receive a free copy of "Yoga and Meditation" can be found in any of my Kindle eBooks.

NOTES

NOTES

NOTES

NOTES

NOTES

NOTES

NOTES

www.ingramcontent.com/pod-product-compliance
Lightning Source LLC
Chambersburg PA
CBHW071009180526
45168CB00003B/1347

* 9 7 8 1 5 1 7 1 2 1 9 2 1 *